The Food Adventure Book

The Food Adventure Book

Changing Your Thinking One Bite at a Time

Kathleen T. Regan, Ph.D.

This book is dedicated to my granddaughter, Emma Kathleen, who inspired me to develop ways to encourage proper nutrition for optimum health for all children.

There is no greater joy than teaching our children to live life well with proper eating, proper resting, proper exercise, and proper thinking.

"The Paths Are Many; the Truth Is One."

"Serve, Love, Give, Purify, Meditate, Realize."

Gratitude to All My Teachers of Light.

I gratefully acknowledge the faith and support
given me by the following people:

My mother Theresa V. Regan, grandmother Vincenza Galgano,
Dr. David Rothblat, Dr. Mahavir Chaturvedi, Julie Kaplan,
Alison Gilbert, Elaine Dale, Robert Shanley, Lester Packer,
Gale Saumya Lichter, Anne Williams, Marguerite Jhonson,
Dr. Karen Engelman, Stuart Paris and Joseph H. Gelberman, Ph.D.

Special Thanks to:
Editor Lynne Matous for her dedication, insight, and wisdom.

Illustrator Phillip Jacobs for his keen imagination, dedication, and skill.

May the Whole World Attain Peace,
Health, Happiness and Love

Goals of *The Food Adventure Book*

To encourage, educate, and enlighten our children about right and proper eating habits for optimum health and to be fully alive. Objectives:

• Encourage children to try the taste of nutritious new foods.

• Motivate children to try a new healthy food with an entry of words, pictures, and drawings in *The Food Adventure Book.*

• Reinforce the eating or tasting of a particular nutritious food by reading *The Food Adventure Book* to the child after the individual chapters and the book are complete.

• Educate children about proper eating habits and proper nutrition. Educate children about respecting and taking care of their body temple.

• Allow children to teach other family members and friends about good healthy eating habits.

• Encourage children to draw and color organic forms from observation.

• Encourage children to read, write, and count.

• Strengthen the right side of the brain by drawing and assembling collages.

• Encourage the ability to make healthy and wise choices.

Joseph H. Gelberman, Ph.D.
Ingredients for a Healthy Life

L I F E

"L" Love unconditionally
"I" Inspire unconditionally
"F" Forgive unconditionally
"E" Eat foods that are alive
(Be excited unconditionally)

A L I V E

"A" Acknowledge that God is my source
"L" Live fully conscious
"I" Innovative thinking
"V" Victorious being
"E" Enthusiastic living

My Favorite Fruits

Apples are healthy.
Oranges rule.
Berries and cherries
are tasty and cool.
Figs are fantastic.
Kiwi is sweet.
Mangos and melons
are surely a treat.
Peaches are scrumptious.
Pears are delicious.
Plums and bananas
are fun and nutritious.
These are the fruits
that I like to devour,
but lemons and grapefruits
are bitter and sour!

By Darren Sardelli

Cupid's Arrow

When I was in the lunchroom,
eating pumpkin pie,
Cupid shot an arrow
that hit me in the thigh.

I looked up at the ceiling
and saw him with his bow.
He took a second arrow
and shot me in the toe.

Another arrow struck me
and knocked me off my seat.
I felt a happy tingle,
which made me shake my feet.

I landed on an apple.
The apple looked so cute.
I simply cannot help it-
I'm now in love with FRUIT!

by Darren Sardelli

Introduction for Parents

For ages parents globally have been struggling to get their children to eat and drink healthy foods and beverages. In addition to using subterfuge, parents have had to coax, cajole, threaten, scold, and beg little ones to eat healthy and nutritious foods — rarely with success and mostly with failure. All parents want their children to eat nutritious foods for optimal health; however, getting children to eat healthy foods is not always that simple.

Young children often have various reactions to food choices. Some feel they want only white food; some like their food separated. Other children will eat only foods that are not mushy or foods that are not too dry. Some children will eat only three items of food, and the list goes on and on. Parents usually fall short in their efforts to feed their children foods with adequate vitamins, minerals, trace minerals, fatty acids, plant nutrients, and fiber because of several factors: the pickiness of their children's eating habits, power struggles, and competition from the unhealthy processed foods their children desire.

During the 1960's the cartoon "*Popeye the Sailor Man*" helped to encourage children to eat spinach. The cartoon's hero, Popeye, reached for his can of spinach whenever he needed a physical and/or mental boost. The consumption of just one can enabled him to accomplish superhuman feats and overcome impossible conditions. Children in the 1960's loved to imitate Popeye the Sailor Man and eat spinach.

Unfortunately, far too little is taught to young children about the benefits of good nutrition and healthy food choices and their relationship to becoming healthy adults. Children have poor perception when it comes to looking down the road into adulthood. Children do not realize that when the body does not get enough nutrients a deficiency or shortage occurs. The symptoms or effects depend on the severity of the deficiency. The early signs of deficiency, however, may not show as something serious or noticeable. Such signs may include tiredness, difficulty in sleeping or concentrating, mood swings, frequent colds, and weight gain or weight loss. Perhaps with the understanding that wise food choices will make them smarter, healthier, stronger, better at sports, and even prettier, their interest in good nutrition may be sparked.

What impact do the junk food, processed food, and chemically impregnated foods have on your child's brain and, therefore, learning ability? Although brain cells are strong cells created to perform even in adverse conditions, how well the brain performs depends on the quality of the nutrients it receives. Chemically laden, processed, sugary, or over-salty foods are perceived by the brain as toxic substances and as stress that inhibits peak performance.

Additionally, the chronic ear and throat infections suffered by many young children are related to the types of foods they eat. For example, research has shown a profound connection between chronic ear infections and the consumption of dairy products. Parents who intend the best for their children need to be aware of the relationship between food and chronic childhood allergies and illnesses. Educating both parents and children concerning which foods to eat and which foods to avoid can have a major impact on their children's overall health now and later in life. Such education is especially important since childhood obesity, diabetes, and cardiovascular diseases are on the rise in the United States, foreshadowing the sprouting of these same diseases, including cancer, in adults. Together both parents and children can make simple, healthy changes in their dietary lifestyles one food at a time, thereby avoiding childhood and adult obesity, while lessening the risk of some life-threatening diseases.

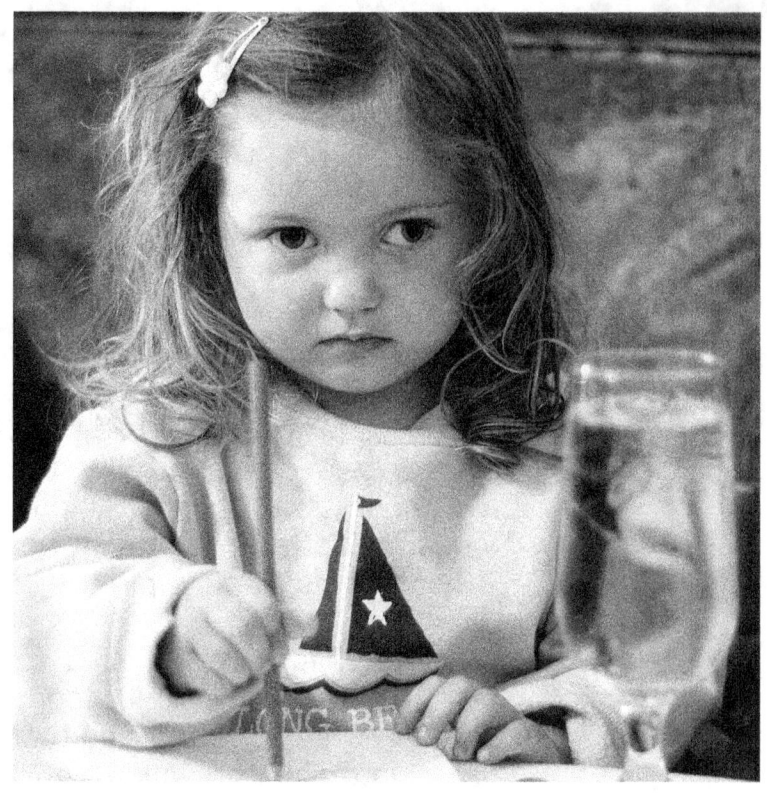

Emma Kathleen Rickert

Knowledge concerning the ingredients in the foods we eat is also vitally important to maintaining good health. Junk foods (including deep fried foods) and junk drinks that are filled with chemicals, hydrogenated fat, corn syrup, high fructose, and sugar are toxins to the brains of young children. Eating such unhealthy, toxin-filled foods can result in learning and behavior problems in children. Sadly, the toxic foods just described are the junk foods that most kids are eating today.

Unfortunately for the health of today's children, the media and marketing "geniuses" have created food and beverage package designs to appeal to young minds for the purpose of increasing sales. The attractive, clever package designs have eye-catching colors and shapes. They present super heroes, cartoon characters, princesses, movie stars, and sports figures to subliminally attract young minds. Therefore, it is important to read labels and educate your children to read labels too. This label-reading can become a game of sorts when shopping in the grocery stores.

Reading labels, however, will not reveal the whole story. Sadly, today's fruits, vegetables, poultry, fish, and dairy (unless raised or grown organically) are routinely sprayed and contaminated with chemical fertilizers and pesticides, and/or injected with hormones. The justification for the use of these harmful chemicals is to speed up growth, increase size, and/or delay ripening of fruits and vegetables. Additionally, to enhance the appearance of fresh vegetables and fruits, they are "polished" with wax, shellac, and dyes.

Be keenly observant when purchasing prepared baked goods boxed or wrapped in plastic. Read the labels carefully. If you spy chemicals that are injurious to human health reconsider this purchase. White flour (usually the primary ingredient) has been stripped of the nutritious part of the seed, removing the bran and wheat germ. Chlorine gases are used to bleach the flour to make it pure white. Then the flour is enriched with synthetic versions of some of the nutrients that were removed. Ever WONDER why certain white breads and boxed cakes will stay for weeks without spoiling and green molding? To add additional flavor and increase shelf life, a host of chemicals are include to these baked goods, such as corn syrup, chlorine dioxide, benzoyl peroxide, acetone peroxide, and in some case, plaster of Paris.

Now the question (addressed by this book) arises — how can we get our kids to make healthy food choices when we are in competition with the colorful visually appealing fast food industry? The fast food restaurants selling the heavily-advertised, highly processed industrial foods (as described above) are the ones that our children are drawn to the most and the ones that they should avoid. Unfortunately, 99% of these appealingly-packaged convenience, often bio-engineered "frankenfoods" (laden with fat, sugar, salt, artificial colors, and chemicals most adults can-

not pronounce) are ultimately injurious to one's optimal health. There have been numerous studies concerning the negative effects of red and blue dyes on children's behavior.

From the early age of toddlers, children are the prime targets for marketing and advertising gimmicks for the purpose of financial gain. Displaying eye-catching visual elements children desire, the manufacturers' clever packaging gimmicks are quite effective in capturing the attention of young minds. Sadly, the manufacturers of these foods have little regard for the nutritional value of the items packaged for children, and parents too often lose the battle when trying to prevail against their clever arsenal of gimmicks.

Like most children, my granddaughter, Emma, is impressed with visual elements of food packaging. She often verbalizes her desires while shopping in the supermarket or asking to go to a fast food restaurant.

In 2009 while we were visiting a Yoga Ashram in New York, another guest noticed me struggling to get my granddaughter Emma to try the wholesome vegetarian food being served. She suggested I motivate Emma to eat nutritious foods by starting a notebook where Emma could list the name and draw the picture of any healthy new food she would try. I immediately embraced this concept and developed Emma's first **Food Adventure Book** out of construction paper, crayons, stickers, and markers.

Amazing results happen.....
Over the next two years the **Food Adventure Book** became the motivating factor encouraging Emma to venture out and try new healthy foods. Her first **Food Adventure Book** had "chapters" on kale, mango, squash, red peppers, water with fresh mint, quinoa, Indian dahl, and more. I noticed that Emma would repeatedly eat

the nutritious foods that appeared in the **Food Adventure Book** with no prodding or cajoling. The purpose of this book is to help you motivate and educate your children to eat nutritious foods that lead to optimum health.

While many children experience immense fear and resistance when faced with having to eat a new foreign food (especially if the food is green), making a game out of eating new, healthy food items can overcome their fear of food they perceive as new, bad tasting, or different. Also, children who are known as "picky eaters" may respond more positively to a description of what a "new" food will taste like. Rather than merely saying, "Try this. It's healthy," say, "Try this food. It tastes sweet (or creamy)."

Creating the chapters in the **Food Adventure Book** can be a stimulating, rewarding and fun family activity. The children will be motivated to try just one bite, knowing that they can create a new chapter in their **Food Adventure Book**. Improve their health one bite at a time.

When the chapters are filled, they become a fun book from which to read and learn. Also, you can discuss the events that surrounded the trying of a particular food making the chapter nostalgic. Children can share their **Food Adventure Book** with their friends, school mates, cousins, and siblings. Parents can reinforce the new foods tried in this workbook by going to a children's library and checking out books on food, farming, anatomy, botany, and nutrition. Children will learn to read words; identify colors and textures; and draw many fruits, vegetables, and shapes. Also, reading their **Food Adventure Book** reinforces the eating of these foods again and again without much, if any, coaching.

Children can be shown where the food goes after it enters their mouths and where their intestines are located. Also, a field trip to a local produce market, farmers market, or health food store will reinforce and motivate healthy eating habits. Taking children to a farm or garden and showing them how fruits, vegetables, and grains are grown can prove invaluable to their connection with eating fresh produce.

Additionally, children experience "hands-on" how a book is developed one chapter at a time. As they create their own book, they can add stickers, color in the background, add silly characters, and let their imaginations go wild. As an added plus, you may notice your child's increased desire to read books in general.

Creating and reading their own **Food Adventure Book**, children learn "by doing" that the choices they make about food affect their total health: body, mind, and spirit. The right, or nutritious, food choices they make (and record in their **Food Adventure Book**) will have a positive impact on the way they think, play, and learn. Eating properly will have a positive impact on their overall behavior, health, and ability to focus and learn in school. Keep in mind that the foods your children eat can be nutritious and simple to prepare; complicated recipes are not necessary for eating healthily. Praise your child often for every effort and most of all have fun exploring new tastes as an adventure in the game of life.

How to Use This Book

A. Motivate

First, talk about the **Food Adventure Book** with your child. Encourage your child to become excited about eating healthily and about creating his or her own book. Explain in simple terms what fat, refined sugar, salt, vitamins and minerals are and why is it important to eat foods that are rich in vitamins and minerals. Then select a healthy food you would like your child to try.

Example: carrots
Q. What are carrots?
A. Carrots are a low calorie, nutritious root vegetable that grows under the ground with its green leaves growing above the ground towards the sun. Carrots taste great, are low in calories, and make an excellent snack food. Carrots come in a variety of colors: orange, yellow, purple, white, and red.

Now, show your child a picture of a carrot or draw a carrot or have your child draw a carrot. You may show your child a real carrot to hold and feel. Explain that carrots can be cooked or eaten raw. Use a potato peeler to peel the outer layer and then peel one layer for your child to eat. Sometimes when offering a child a "new" raw vegetable, a thin peel may be more appealing than a thick slice.

Now show your child the **Food Adventure Book** and explain how a food qualifies for the book even if it is only one taste of a new food choice. Then, after eating a bit of raw carrot, your child may draw and color a picture of a carrot in the book. You can add to the fun by doing activities suggested in this book and further educate your child by discussing such topics as vitamins, minerals, nutrients, and phytochemicals — pointing out the ones that are in carrots. Then you or your child can add (under the picture of carrots) the names of the vitamins and minerals that are found in this vegetable (Vitamins: A, B1, B2, B5, B6, K; phytochemicals: carotenoid; minerals: potassium, phosphorus, calcium).

Let your child fill in the chapter names and descriptions, or if your child is too young to write, you can write in the names of the food, while teaching your child the letters for each food's name.

Each completed chapter can be read over and over to reinforce reading, phonics, spelling, and visual memory, in addition to reinforcing the consumption and taste of that particular food. Thus, each completed chapter becomes a mini-lesson in cognitive learning, art, crafts, reading, writing, botany, nutrition, and science.

B. Further guidelines for using the Food Adventure Book

1. Gather pictures, stickers, and stamps of healthy foods, together with crayons and markers.

2. When your child tries a new healthy food have the book and supplies nearby ready to reward the child with his or her first chapter.

3. Work with one food at a time. It will be more effective to isolate one food at a time.

4. Write the name of the food as the title for a chapter in the Table of Contents, starting with "Chapter One."

5. Title the first page of the chapter with the name of the food.

6. Draw the food or glue a picture of the food onto the page.

7. Embellish the picture and page with colors, stickers, stamps, or collages.

8. Frequently talk about and read the **Food Adventure Book** with your child. This reinforces the value and benefits of eating healthy foods and avoiding ones that are unhealthy.

9. Stress the benefits of eating fresh vegetables, fruits, and whole grain breads, while avoiding foods that have high fat and caloric content. (A diet with increased caloric intake, such as highly processed fast food, is one cause of an increased incidence of cancer. Science has shown us through hundreds of studies that a decrease in the consumption of fat and highly caloric foods can reduce the chances of later developing tumors and prostate, colon, breast, endometrial, and ovarian cancers.)

10. Have fun trying a variety of healthy foods, by making an adventure spin dial game board to help your child decide what food to pick for the day. Make the categories fruits, vegetables, grains, nuts, seeds, proteins and legumes.

Summary

The Food Adventure Book has provided a creative, safe and fun way to encourage and educate your child to eat right. The knowledge you have gained herein will enable you to encourage your child to try new healthy foods and adopt a healthier life style. You have learned that adopting a diet filled with pure and natural foods will provide the body with the essential vitamins, minerals, and nutrients to sustain a healthy life. In other words, eating right for optimum health can give you and your child the power to begin to shape your future health. Lastly, this book was written to help parents and their children incorporate beneficial foods into their daily diet and avoid unhealthy foods that are a prescription for future disease. Kids willingly and repeatedly eat the foods in their **Food Adventure Book.**

Glossary

Fruits: the ripened fleshy form of a seed bearing plant; apples, grapes, plums, tomatoes, peppers.

GMO: genetically modified organisms and foods.

Grains: a small dry, one-seeded fruit of a cereal grass.

Herbs: any of various aromatic plants used in medicine, tea, or cooking. Examples: basil, catnip, chives, lemon grass, oregano, peppermint.

Hydrogenated Oils: brain-toxic, altered fat; hydrogenation is a process where hydrogen is pumped into the oil molecules at high temperatures turning vegetable oil into thick heat resistant saturated fat.

Junk Drinks: sugary, drinks made from corn syrup, high fructose, sugar, artificial flavors and colors, and chemical food contaminants.

Junk Food: foods high in calories, fat, sugar, and salt; processed, chemical preservatives, artificial colors and flavors, and sometimes food contaminants are added.

Legume: Dry beans, nuts, lentils, peanuts, and peas are complementary proteins. This means each supplies amino acids that the other lacks. For example, beans and rice are complementary proteins, as are whole grain bread and nut butter.

Nutrient: a nourishing ingredient in food.

Mineral: an inorganic element, such as calcium, essential to the nutrition of human beings, animals, and plants.

Salt: a granulated mineral that is added to food to give taste and zest.

Saturated fats: fats that are solid at room temperature; found in animal foods such as meats, poultry, egg yolks, and whole milk dairy products.

Sour: having a taste that is tart, sharp, or tangy.

Unsaturated fats: fats that are usually liquid at room temperature found in vegetable oils, with the exception of tropical oils (palm and coconut).

Vegetable: a plant cultivated for an edible part containing minerals, vitamins and fiber. Examples: beets, carrots, celery, kale, lettuce, parsnips.

Vitamins: any of various fat or water soluble organic substances essential for growth and health derived from plants or animals. Examples: vitamin A, C, D.

Tips and Tidbits

- Respect your food. Begin each meal by giving thanks for it.
- Make dietary changes slowly. Do not force your child to try a new food. Entice your child with a happy smile and with a food that is colorful and visually appealing.
- Enjoy mealtime with your family. Turn off TV's, cell phones, tablets, computer, and handheld video games.
- End the moaning and groaning of forcing healthy food on your child by maintaining a pleasant and peaceful attitude during meals.
- Try easy recipes to entice your child to experiment and participate in simple, age appropriate cooking.
- Make a colorful apron with pictures of fruits, vegetables, and herbs that your child can wear while cooking.
- Try to refrain from drinking during a meal as fluids will dilute gastric juices needed for digestion.
- Eat slowly and chew thoroughly, remembering that digestion begins in the mouth.
- Add smashed fresh fruits to plain cream cheese or yogurt.
- Make your own toasted granola with oats, nuts, seeds, and maple syrup.
- Try carob as a chocolate alternative. It is rich in natural sugar, calcium, and minerals.
- Go organic!
- Go Green!

- Offer your child a cow milk alternative: organic rice, soy, hemp, oat, or almond milk.
- Create a funny face or animal using fruits, nuts, and seeds.
- Create a funny face , fish, or animal using sliced vegetables, seeds, and nuts.
- Create a healthy salad dressing or vegetable dip in a blender or food processor — there are endless recipes and ingredients for homemade salad dressings. The basics should include fresh lime, grapefruit, or lemon, olive oil, and a drop of tamari or soy sauce. If you wish, add one or more of these natural ingredients: seeds, nuts, carrots, beets, cucumber, tomatoes, radishes, parsley, cilantro, dill, tahini sauce (sesame seed paste high in vitamin E), nut butter, mint, mustard, or yogurt.
- Eat fresh food. Avoid stale, old, tasteless, burnt, fried, reheated (many times), undercooked, overcooked, processed, rotten, and preserved food.
- Store nuts and seeds in the freezer to maintain freshness and avoid rancidity.
- Deep fried foods are indigestible; try to avoid them.
- Make Nori rolls filled with cooked rice and thinly sliced vegetables. Nori is high in protein, vitamins A and B1, kelp and trace minerals. It is also a good source of iodine.
- Use natural sweeteners: stevia, honey, apple juice concentrate, barley malt, syrup, molasses, maple syrup, sucanat and agave nectar. Avoid white sugar, high fructose corn syrup and artificial sweeteners in pink or blue packets.
- Add Miso (a cultured paste made from soy beans, rice, or barley) to soups and sauces. Miso is high in protein and vitamin B12.
- Use fresh ingredients, whenever possible. Limit use of thawed or canned foods.
- Cold Herbal teas can be sweetened with stevia, grape or apple juice,

making a healthy alternative to soda and sugary juice drinks.

- Introduce your child to freshly squeezed fruits and vegetable juices.
- Have kids create a rainbow on their plates by choosing an assortment of fresh colorful foods.
- Use cilantro in your food for added Vit C, Vit K, vision-enhancing carotenoids, and compounds that reduce Alzheimer's symptoms and cholesterol.
- Try making organic baby food for your infant or toddler. Cook a sweet potato, add some water or broth, blend in a food processor, store in small glass jars, and refrigerate; good for 2-3 days.
- Create numbers and alphabet letters by using berries and small pieces of other fruits and vegetables to form shapes of letters and numbers. Young children can form letters; older children can create their name, favorite word, and birthday, also their address, phone number, etc.
- Eat Honey. A spoonful a day strengthens the immune system. Honey is the only food on earth that will not spoil or rot. Never boil honey or put it in a microwave; it will kill the enzymes. Honey taken with some cinnamon aids the immune system: clears sinuses, helps cure colds, sore throats, and influenza..
- Surround your family with healthy foods.
- Keep a platter of such healthy snacks as apple slices, organic seeds, nuts, and cheese and vegetable match sticks, curls, or slices where your kids can reach them.
- If your kids crave junk food try popping corn and adding flavors like grated cheese. Never give a child five year or younger popcorn, as they can easily choke.

Suggested Websites and Readings

www.kidshealth.org

www.mealsmatter.org

www.nutritionforkids.com

Charmine, Susan E. **The Complete Raw Juice Therapy**. England: Thorsons Publishers, Ltd., 1977.

Daulter, Anni. **Organically Raised**. Rodale, 2010.

Ewald, Ellen Buchman. **Recipes for a Small Planet**. New York: Ballentine Books, 1973.

Furhman, M.D., Joel. **Eat To Live**. Boston, MA: Little, Brown and Company, 2003.

Green, M.D., Alan. **Feeding Baby Green**. San Francisco, CA: Jossey-Bass, 2009.

Karmel, Annabel. **The Healthy Baby Meal Planner.** New York: Fireside, Simon and Schuster, 1992.

Lyon, M.D., Michael R. **Is Your Child's Brain Starving?** Mind Publishing Inc., 2002.

May, James A. **The Miracle of Stevia: Discover the Healing Power of Nature's Herbal Sweetener.** New York: Kensington Publishing Corp, 2003.

Robbins, John. **Diet for a New America.** Walpole, NH: Stillpoint Publishing, 1987.

The Yoga Vegetarian Cookbook. Fireside, NY: The Sivananda Vedanta Centers, 1999.

Wansink, Brian. **Mindless Eating, Why We Eat More Than We Think**. New York: Bantam Books, 2010.

This *Food Adventure Book*

Belongs to: _____

Date: _____

Have your child draw (or photograph) a self-portrait
eating a new healthy food.

Table of Contents
Write the name of one food for each chapter

Chapter 1

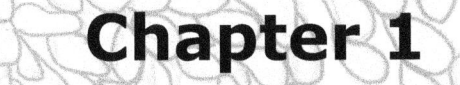

_____

What does the food taste like? _____

What color is it? _____

What texture is it? _____

Chapter 2

_____

What does the food taste like? _____

What color is it? _____

What texture is it? _____

Chapter 3

_____

What does the food taste like? _____

What color is it? _____

What texture is it? _____

Chapter 4

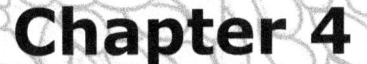

What does the food taste like? _____

What color is it? _____

What texture is it? _____

Chapter 5

_____

What does the food taste like? _____

What color is it? _____

What texture is it? _____

Chapter 6

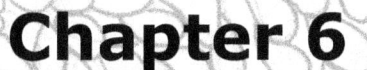

_____

What does the food taste like? _____

What color is it? _____

What texture is it? _____

Chapter 7

_____

What does the food taste like? _____

What color is it? _____

What texture is it? _____

Chapter 8

_____

What does the food taste like? _____

What color is it? _____

What texture is it? _____

Chapter 9

_____

What does the food taste like? _____

What color is it? _____

What texture is it? _____

Chapter 10

_____

What does the food taste like? _____

What color is it? _____

What texture is it? _____

Chapter 11

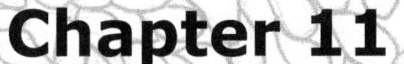

_____

What does the food taste like? _____

What color is it? _____

What texture is it? _____

Chapter 12

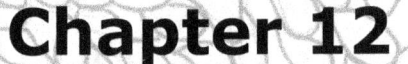

_____

What does the food taste like? _____

What color is it? _____

What texture is it? _____

Chapter 13

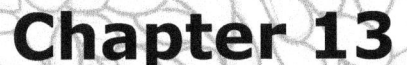

_____

What does the food taste like? _____

What color is it? _____

What texture is it? _____

Chapter 14

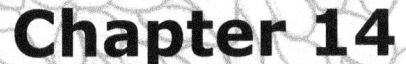

_____

What does the food taste like? _____

What color is it? _____

What texture is it? _____

Chapter 15

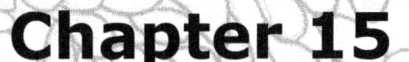

_____

What does the food taste like? _____

What color is it? _____

What texture is it? _____

Chapter 16

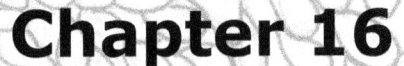

_____

What does the food taste like? _____

What color is it? _____

What texture is it? _____

Chapter 17

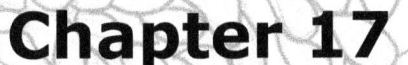

_____

What does the food taste like? _____

What color is it? _____

What texture is it? _____

Chapter 18

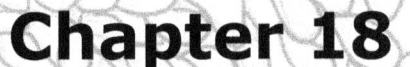

_____

What does the food taste like? _____

What color is it? _____

What texture is it? _____

Chapter 19

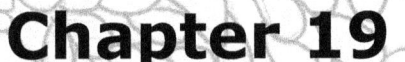

What does the food taste like? _____

What color is it? _____

What texture is it? _____

Chapter 20

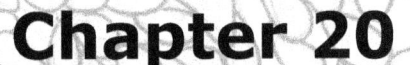

_____

What does the food taste like? _____

What color is it? _____

What texture is it? _____

Chapter 21

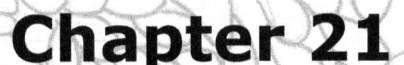

_____

What does the food taste like? _____

What color is it? _____

What texture is it? _____

Chapter 22

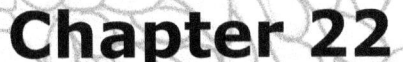

_____

What does the food taste like? _____

What color is it? _____

What texture is it? _____

Chapter 23

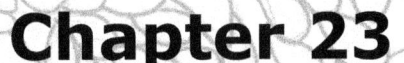

_____

What does the food taste like? _____

What color is it? _____

What texture is it? _____

Chapter 24

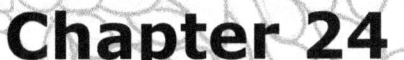

_____

What does the food taste like? _____

What color is it? _____

What texture is it? _____

Chapter 25

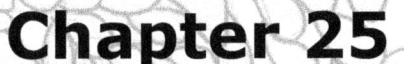

_____

What does the food taste like? _____

What color is it? _____

What texture is it? _____

Chapter 26

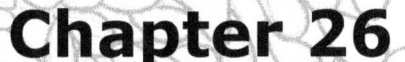

_____

What does the food taste like? _____

What color is it? _____

What texture is it? _____

Chapter 27

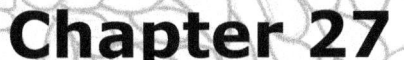

_____

What does the food taste like? _____

What color is it? _____

What texture is it? _____

Chapter 28

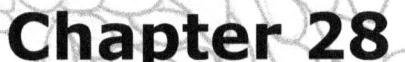

_____

What does the food taste like? _____

What color is it? _____

What texture is it? _____

Chapter 29

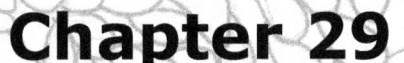

_____

What does the food taste like? _____

What color is it? _____

What texture is it? _____

Chapter 30

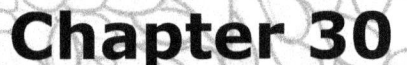

_____

What does the food taste like? _____

What color is it? _____

What texture is it? _____

Recipes I Like

Dear Friends,

Cooking and eating healthy is an adventure as you will find out when you use this book. When you complete this book it will be your unique food and recipe book.

When Emma was 4 she expressed great interest in cooking. So I taught her simple recipes that she had fun making and eating. Emma especially enjoyed making cakes, shakes, and salads. Remember to ask a family member or older adult to assist you when you plan to prepare and cook a special recipe.

You may want to ask a family member for traditional family recipes that your grandparents or aunts and uncles cooked. Children love to hear the stories about their family ancestors through the lens of cooking and family gatherings. Learning about old family recipes is a great way to learn about your family and keep traditions going. Cooking together can be fun and an exciting way to learn favorite family recipes.

On the blank recipe pages write your favorite recipe and then draw and color a picture of what it looks like.. An option can be to take a photo and glue down the print to the bottom of the page.

Always wash your hands and wash the surface of your counter and cutting board before you begin to cook. Rinse all the fruits and vegetables before you begin your recipe.

Most of all remember that you are what you eat. When you eat wisely and healthy you will feel good, have lots of energy, and be strong .

Health is wealth ,Eating right shows you the way. Bon appétit!

Kathleen and Emma

Recipes I Like

What I Will Make: *Raspberry Zing Herbal Ice Tea*

Serves: 4   Cooking time: 5 min.   Preparation time: 10min.

Be sure to ask permission and help from a family member before you cook.

What I will Need?

3 1/2 cups water
1/2 cup grape juice
4 tea bags raspberry zinger tea
1 quart container

What I Will Do?

In large pot boil 4 water. add 4 tea bags; let steep. cover and turn off stove.

Let cool. Add 1/2 cup grape juice; add ice and drink or chill.

Optional: squeeze 1/2 lemon or lime for tart flavor and added Vitamin C You can double the recipe to make more tea.

Draw how does it look like or take a photo and paste it on the space below

Recipes I Like

What I Will Make: Carrot Curls

Serves: **4   Cooking time: None   Preparation time: 20min.**

Be sure to ask permission and help from a family member before you cook.

What I will Need?

4 raw carrots
15 toothpicks
Bowl of ice water

What I Will Do?

Peel fresh crisp carrots with a peeler. Slice the length of carrot paper thin, with a peeler, for long very thin slices.
Roll up each slice around your finger and hold it together with a tooth-pick. Be sure the shape is round. Soak curls in ice water for about 1 hour to hold their shape. Remove from water, put curls on platter and serve.

Draw how does it look like or take a photo and paste it on the space below

Recipes I Like

What I Will Make: Ants on a Log

Serves: 4   Cooking time: 15 min.   Preparation time: 10min.

Be sure to ask permission and help from a family member before you cook.

What I will Need?

4 washed celery stalks
1/2 cup natural nut butter
(any nut butter of your choice)
1/2 cup raisins

What I Will Do?

Wash and Dry the celery ribs. Fill each with nut butter. Place a row of raisins in the middle of each celery rib.   Eat or chill.

Draw how does it look like or take a photo and paste it on the space below

Recipes I Like

What I Will Make: _____

Serves: ___   **Cooking time:** ____min.   **Preparation time:** ____min.

Be sure to ask permission and help from a family member before you cook.

What I will Need?

| |
| |
| |
| |

What I Will Do?

Recipes I Like

What I Will Make: _____

Serves: ___   **Cooking time:** ____min.   **Preparation time:** ____min.

Be sure to ask permission and help from a family member before you cook.

What I will Need?

What I Will Do?

About the Author

I am the grandmother of a 6-year-old girl who has shown me how to teach her to eat healthfully. The experience of raising my granddaughter and teaching her to eat health-fully has been so special, unique, and exciting that I was called to share this book with all the parents and children of the world.

I have been a teacher of children all my life and have seen the sad results of poor eating habits and lack of exercise in our youth. There is now an epidemic of childhood obesity, diabetes, high blood pressure, learning disabilities, mental illness and emotional issues — much of which could be resolved or eliminated by proper and better nutrition. This workbook provides an impetus for families to work together in a fun and healthy way to improve their nutritional intake and their health.

I would love to hear from anyone who has used this workbook to encourage their chil-dren to eat a varied, healthy diet. Additionally, I would like to hear from anyone who has constructive suggestions or information that would be helpful for a future revised edition of this book. It is and always will be my goal for **The Food Adventure Book** to be a great source of encouragement and information to help raise the awareness of our youth concerning eating right for life.

You can contact me at: thefoodadventurebook@gmail.com
and on Face book: The Food Adventure Book.

If you would like to contact the illustrator of this book, Phillip Jacobs, visit www.artbyphiljacobs.com or contact him at: philsart2000@yahoo.com.

—NOTES—

—NOTES—